BALD IN THE MERDE

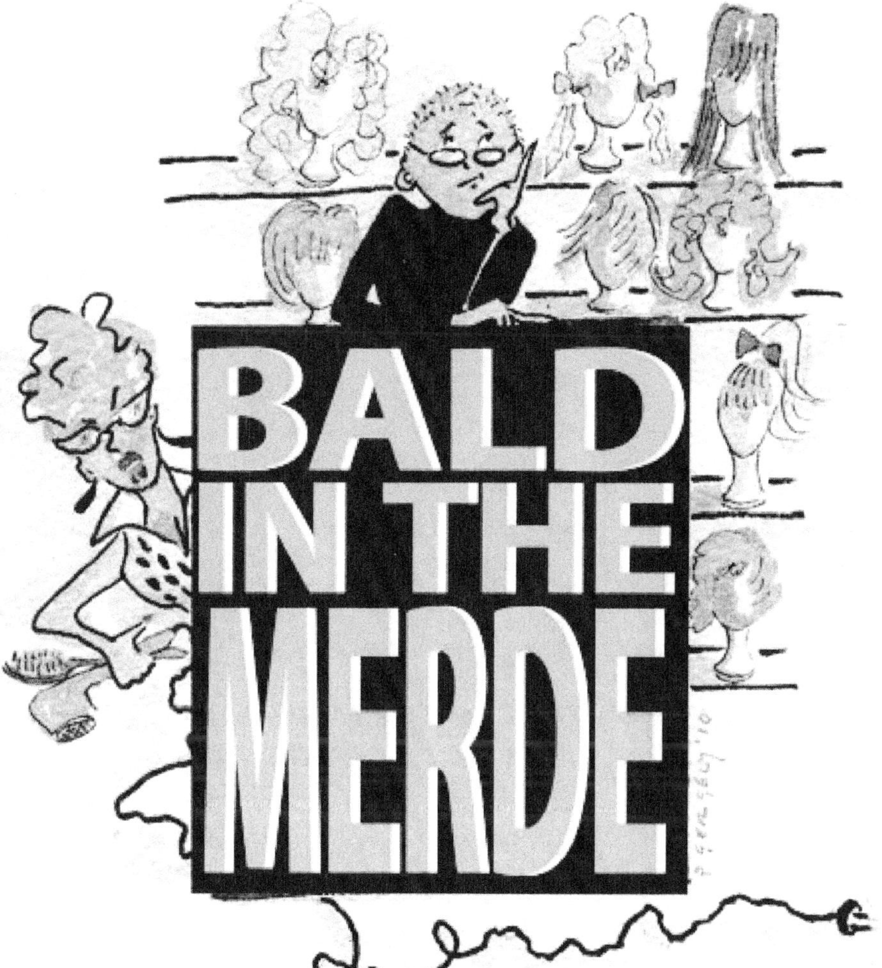

Story by SUZANNE WHITE
Illustrations by PETE GERGELY

Story by SUZANNE WHITE
Illustrated by PETER GERGELY
© suzannewhite/petegergely 2010

all rights reserved

Suzanne White, 38 Miller Avenue, #164, Mill Valley, CA, 94941, USA

http://www.suzannewhite.com

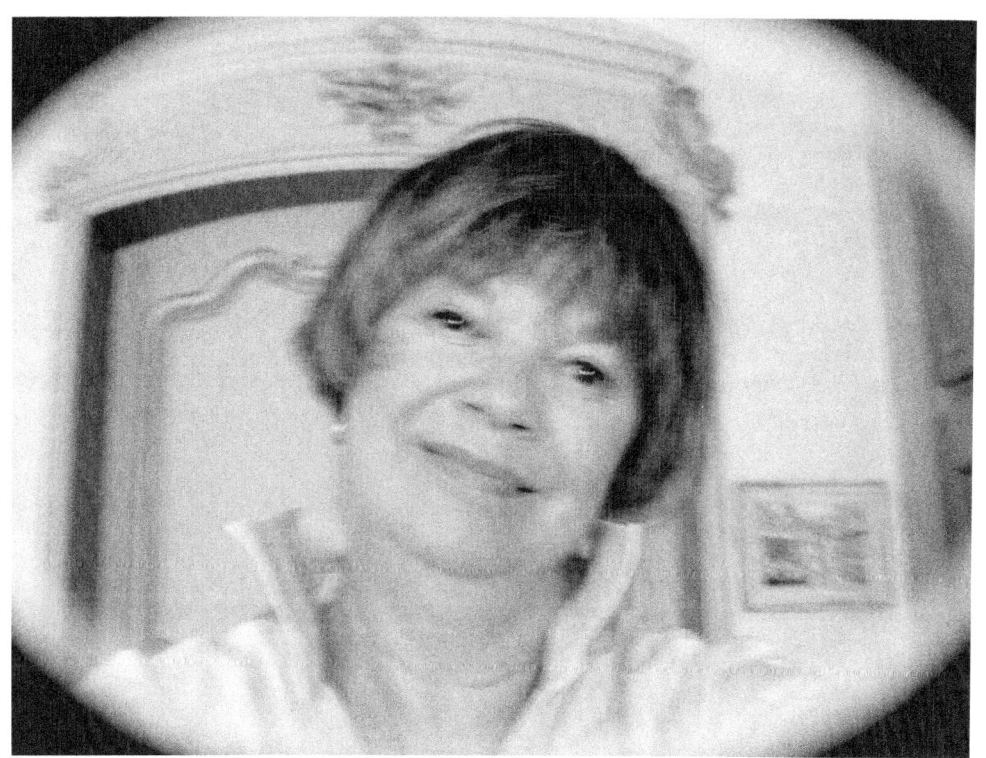

Author Suzanne White be-wigged

DEDICATION

This book is dedicated to every person who helped me get through this, my third cancer journey. I begin with my old friend Dr. Daniel Andreozzi who introduced me to my friend and family physician Dr. Christine Bodo who, in turn, sent me next day to my newfound pal, Dr. Serge Boyer the handsome gray-haired surgeon who removed the tumor along with my
hysteria and saved my life in one fell six-hour swoop of the scalpel.

From then on, I was chemotherapized by Dr. Emmanuel Guardiola, a 39 year old bespectacled oncologist cutey with a laugh that shakes his whole body. While I was being poisoned for 4 or 5 hours 6 different times at 3 week intervals, Emmanuel was my co-conspirator. He slipped me his personal secret code for hospital wifi and brought mt cookies his wife had baked. So even though I was obliged to sit still and let the toxic products drip into my veins, I could work on my laptop, bring my Kindle and/or books and listen to my iPod as well. Emmanuel came by every hour or so to check on me and make me laugh.

My heartfelt thanks to all kind, sweet nurses and funny nurses' aides in the spanking new cancer unit at the Draguignan hospital. They comforted me, cleaned me up and changed my shirt when I accidentally got up to go to the ladies' without unplugging myself and spilled that wretched chemo goo all over my shirt. (ruined of course). I drove home with a hospital gown over my jeans. I use that gown for a cooking apron now.

I owe my morale's survival of the entire episode to loyal, standup friends: Trinka Von Tscharner and Patricia Simoens and Betsy Brill and Ken Kobre and Christel Chaher and Maïté Clément, Laetitia Roussell Boye and the unflinching Aries/Tiger Claude Lombard who not only came to visit me, but brought me treats and flowers and clean clothes and wooly jackets and funny pj's with bears on them to keep me cozy and sane in the convalescent Clinique des Espérels.

Further, I laud and applaud the staff at La Clinique des Espérels. From the office crew to the medical staff to the cleaning ladies, they all coaxed me through the pain and made me giggle when I hurt most. All of them... every last one of them works for the remarkable French Medical System. Every one of them is salaried. And every one of them is loving and kind and good and comes to my house for dinner when invited.

France has frequently saved my life. See for yourself. Read my autobiography UNMITIGATED GAUL. (work in progress) Discover what miracles can happen to a plain vanilla American girl from Buffalo who went to live in Paris in 1961 and never left. sw

Today I am in love.

With a wig.

Last February, in the provincial city of Draguignan-en-Provence, at the *Institut Capillaire Salon,* located in a 500 year old apartment, one rickety flight up, a woman named Danièle offered me a slew of prosthetic head coverings. Danièle is a thin, brittle lady of 58 whose husband recently defected. She's not on top form. She trembles as she combs the polyester strands of her wigs into suitable *coiffures*. She grooms them. Then she wiggle-slides the wigs, one after the other, down over her customers' bare heads.

It was Tuesday. I was still in residence at the lovely country convalescent *Clinique des Espérels*. I'd been given a morning's furlough to drive my own car to town for appointments. At 9:25 I met Jean, my Draguignan hairdresser, pacing the courtyard in front of his salon, smoking and talking on his cell.

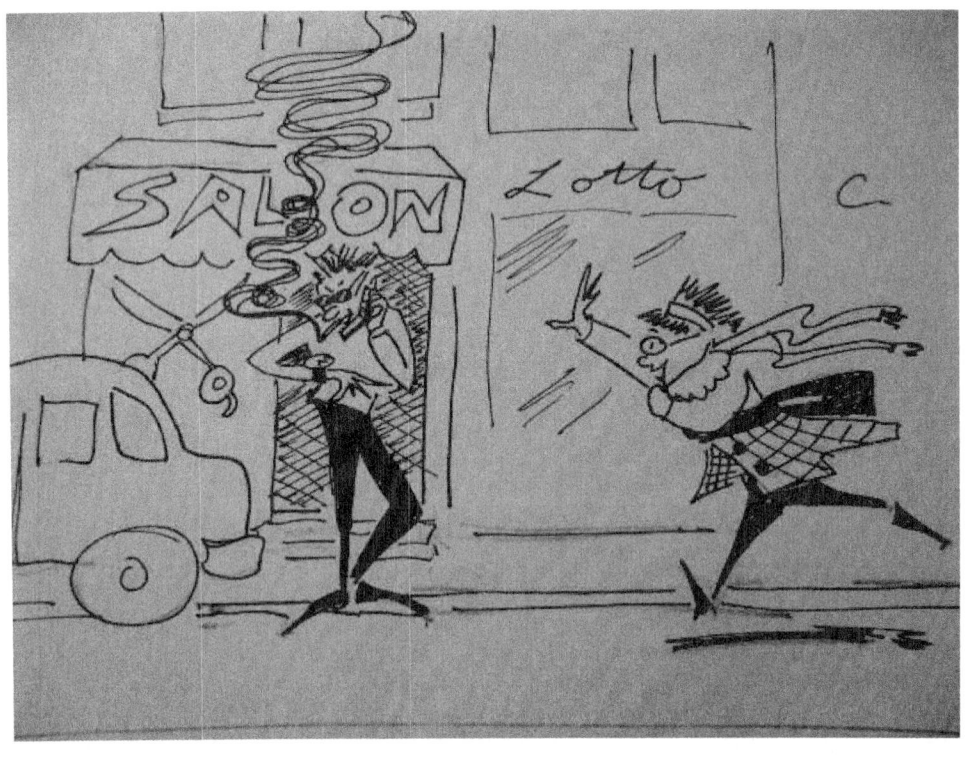

He saw me., ended his phone call, scolded me for being 25 minutes late, put out his cigarette and invited me to come inside. "It's freezing out here." I sat. Jean snipped. As he did so, he nattered on about how we would deal with my *problème.*

Jean Astijiano, my favorite hairdresser, is *Provençal* French, which is not French Provincial. It's *faux* Italian. Jean is Italian the way Al Capone was American. His Italian grandparents emigrated to Provence. So he's French *Provençal* — of Italian descent. Jean has a southern French accent that I can't reproduce here. It hits nasal sounds like the end of the word *matin* (for morning) as though they were made of sheet metal. "Tomorrow morning" (demain matin) sounds like *demaing mataing*. Each word ends with that rattle for which sheet metal is so famous. Jean is a Taurus. In Chinese astrology, Jean is a garrulous Rat. He doesn't talk. He yaks. Rat-a-tat tat. Constantly. "I have a new husband," he whispers in my one ear - *and out the other*. I gaze past my half-bald head in the gilt-framed mirror before me and shudder. The gaudy wall colors reflected there are so distinctively *Draguignan*.

"What's his name?" I must appear curious about Jean's new husband. In 20 years of coming to Jean for all my hair issues, I had waded through a fair number of his conquests and likewise, he mine. We are on familiar verb form terms. "You still think I'm the best hairdresser in Christendom?" he wondered.

"Naturellement," I answered. And it's true. I have lived in Paris, New York, San Francisco and Buenos Aires. Yet here in pokey old Draguignan, which is anything but *chic Provence,* the best hairdresser on the globe, my secret weapon, plies his trade. In Draguignan, there are 74 hairdressers. That's for only 30,000 people. *Big Hair* is everywhere. There's even a hairdresser in Draguignan called *Self Coiffure.* I have often asked myself how that works. Is it like a self-service cafeteria? You put your head on a tray and slide it along a set of smooth metal bars till you reach the sink and then the *Self coiffing* begins? Beats me.

Jean is the Pied Piper of Draguignan hairdressers. He has not always been with the same salon. But whither goest Jean Asitjiano and his magic scissors around this town, the women of *Le Tout Draguignan* slavishly follow.

Poor Draguignan. She is an ancient city with a deep and magical history. Dukes and *Duchesses* - nobles of every stripe and rank danced and daggered through the streets of the old walled city for eons before some clodhopping 20th century politicians tarted it up with monuments to bad taste. Nowadays, awkward sculptures, clumsy statues and dead-in-the water fountains crowd the too many roundabouts where rampaging drivers, rev and *vroom* day and night. It's a busy little city. The farmer's market stalls on Wednesday and Saturdays foam with fresh produce, olive oils, local goat cheeses, multicolored olives and easy-drinking *rosés de Provence.* Draguignan is warm and sunny and convivial. But Paris or New York or San Francisco or Buenos Aires... Draguignan is decidely not.

"His name is Frédéric," said Jean, smiling at me in the mirror. "But I call him Fred." He winked.

"Is he a real husband?" I asked. It was a disingenuous question. "Are you ... married?"

"*Bien sûr que non!* " Jean assured me. "Of course not." Then added, "Anyway, it's against the law."

"Just as well," I replied. "Marriage isn't exactly your style."

Jean laughed out loud. As he doesn't own the chintz-festooned pink
and purple salon where he's working now, I can't hold him responsible for
the garish color scheme. Here at *LaTiffa Coiffures*, Jean is an employee. He
did run his own tastefully overdone red plush and golden-curtained salon
some years back. But when the banker lover split, Jean lost his financing.

He stops snipping, stares at me for a sec and says, "My new husband is
actually kind of chubby. I mean he's big. And strong." Jean holds the
scissors wide open over my head and glances in the mirror at the result of his
work. "Okay. So Fred's a little fat. But he's a nurse's aide. He's so kind. He
loves me. I love him." Jean sucks in some air. "... And he cooks!"

"Maybe you should just shave it off, " I said with a shrug, returning the
subject to what remained of my hair. "What's the use of these spiky tufts?"

"Don't ask me to. I would never shave anyone's head - yes maybe a guy - a
younger gay guy... if he was cute - but you don't shave a woman. Too brutal.
Too shocking. This way the hair still falls out. But it goes gradually. You
know it's going. But because it's so short, it doesn't leave great swarms and
strands on your lover's chest or in the kitchen sink." The skin around Jean's
eyes crinkled. Jean thinks he's funny. I am 71 and currently loverless.

He scissored my hair to half an inch everywhere. I looked like a *tondue,* one
of those French women they sheared bald after the war for having copulated

with a handsome German or three. The color? Blonde and white mixed. Like beer.

Jean charged me 21 euros and urged me hurry on over to the wig salon where I was expected at 10. "Avoid wearing navy blue and black." He said, "Short white hairs show up as dandruff on those colors." I scooted out the door.

I hurried along to the *Insitut Capillaire.* At the top of the stairs, I was welcomed by the stout, odiferous Portuguese cleaning lady who was vacking up the tile floors. Pleasant surprise. She did not smell of the characteristic Portugese *concierge* dried salt cod I had come to know so well in Paris in the 20th century. This cleaning person's fragrance was either Opium by Saint-Laurent or Guerlain's Shalimar. Heady. Dense. It blended effectively with and masked the chemical odor of the tile cleaner in the yellow bucket at her feet.

Sponge mops are not the custom in France. To clean our deep red *Provençal* tiles, you vacuum first and then wash with a large dingy wet waffle-weave rag called a *serpillière* that you first soak in a mixture of super hot water and a commercial tile-cleaning product. Then you pinch up the near-scalding, soaking-wet rag and wrap it loosely around the business end of a brush screwed to a broom handle. To wash and shine the tiles, you swoop this contraption around all the floors. The way you drape the rag around the brush is crucial. You must leave some flaps of the cloth free to thwack about as you swish and swirl across the ceramic floors. Those exposed flapping bits are expected to creep into the crannies of your room of their own volition and lap up the dirt. When you reckon the *serpillère* is filthy enough, you remove it from the brush and dunk it into the bucket a few times. Then you wring it out with your bare hands and whack it back onto the brush-broom gizmo. This novel deck-swabbing system is traditionally used on tiles floors all over France. It works a treat.

"We're cleaning," said the cleaning woman.

I had gathered that, so I stepped gingerly over the bunched wet *serpillière* she'd left on the top step and walked into a small zig-zaggy apartment. A minimal space had been further minimized by breaking it into 2.5 tiny rooms. Whipped cream peaks of plaster held years of gritty dust on the walls. The floor was covered in typical, authentic 500-year-old hexagonal Salernes *tomettes* tiles. Some of the looser tiles clanked and crunched as I walked through the foyer into the shop. "*Bonjour!*" I called out. "*Danièle est là?*"

Danièle came forward and identified herself. "*Je suis Danièle,*" she said.

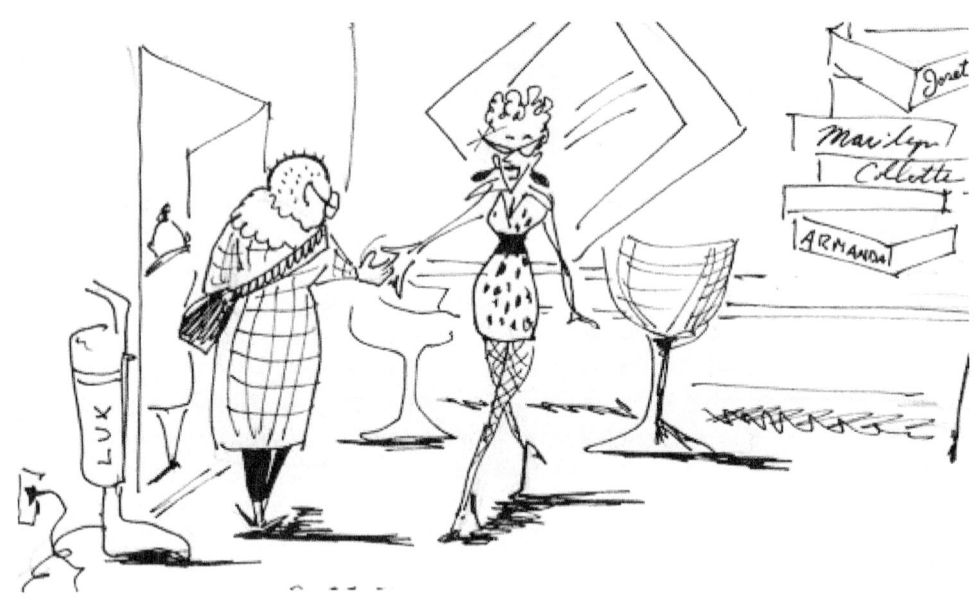

"Bonjour. Je suis Suzanne White."

"Bonjour Madame White," shrilled Danièle. We shook ladylike hands.

We would be just the two of us, she explained. The boss, Pascal, whom I had met the previous Saturday, was fitting wigs in two nearby hospitals. Danièle gestured I should precede her into one of the tiny roomlets, where I settled into a modern design barber chair in front of a skew-gee diamond-shaped mirror.

To my right was a wall of white cardboard shoeboxes. They all had names: Colette, Patty, Juliette, Denise, Marilyn. And color labels: ash blonde, salt and pepper, black pepper, snow white, sandy, auburn and dark brown. Wigs. Hundreds of them lined the walls. It was almost too warm in there. Or was it a hot flash? The noise of the vacuum cleaner made it necessary to shout. I shouted. "I tried on one on Saturday. Pascal told me he would put it aside."

"Oh you must be the Armanda lady," piped Danièle. She flounced off through the door into the front room to find Armanda. The vacuuming ceased. She exchanged some words with the cleaner and wished her "*Courage*!" before bidding her *au revoir*.

While Danièle was out, I took a gander around. Across from me to the left, there was an ancient hair-washing sink. Its plastic leather chair's seat was torn. A free-range red foam cushion failed to conceal the tear. An electrical outlet had exited the wall. It hung midair next to the faucets, with a large black plug pushed inside. An auxiliary heater switched noisily on and off as doors opened and closed, blowing gushes of cooler air at its thermostat. I examined the plugs at ankle level. They, too, had begun to abandon their moorings. The switch for the lights was jiggly, threatening to leap into the void.

Danièle came back with a white box. "Armanda" she said. "It was right there with your name on it." She showed me the Armanda box. "Pascal is more efficient than me," she said, holding the box aloft. On the end ARMANDA was writ large in magic marker. Madame White was scrawled by hand on a fuschia post-it stuck right there. Danièle went on. "Pascal is meticulous. He files everything just where it should go. He has to get after me sometimes. I'm not that organized. Once a woman went home with a man's wig," said Danièle, chuckling. "I put it in the wrong box. Pascal was furious." She blushed. "But he was right. And, Madame White, believe me I don't mean to speak against my boss. He's very clever." Danièle waved a broad gesture around the small room, stretching out her spiny fingers. " Pascal did all the work in here himself. Every bit. The plaster, the plumbing, the electricity. Pascal knows what he's doing. He's a specialist."

Teasing Armanda from the box with her glossy pink fingernails, Danièle gave it a quick comb through, sashayed around behind me and wriggled the wig's elastic border down over my head. It felt a bit like a stocking cap, except the ears stayed out. I looked in the mirror. It seemed fine. Shortish straight, light brown hair with bangs and subtle highlights. Looked just as good as it had on Saturday. "I like this one," I said.

Why did I like it so much? Because the Armanda wig did not look like a wig. Once upon my head, Armanda gave the impression it was the real me with a good blunt cut on straight blondish hair. It looked indeed rather like my own hair before the chemicals murdered it. Shorter. But the same color. The dyed color. Underneath, I suppose I had gray hair. But I don't know that for sure. I must have been about 30 when I began to see white hairs popping up all over in my thick dark brown locks. I lived in Paris then. Gray hairs would not do. For 25 years I had my hair dyed my natural all-over brown to cover the gray. Then, when I was 58, I went to Jean and asked him to dye my hair the routine same brown as usual. I had to dye it often now to cover the increasingly gray roots.

"Please Jean. Make it look natural," said I.

Jean peered around the salon to be sure everyone was paying attention and then shouted, "Madame White just had the best facelift in all of France and she still wants hair the color of a muskrat."

The women all turned. All stared. One squeaky voice said, "That's a facelift?" Another gasped. A third whistled and said, "That's perfect. Give me the name of your surgeon."

Interrupting this hail of shrill remarks, Jean addressed me directly in the mirror, "Why, Suzanne White, on God's earth do you insist on having brown hair? This is *Provence,* Suzanne. The sun shines every day. The sun turns dyed brown hair orange. Do you want orange hair?"

"Certainly not!" I retorted. "But I am used to brown."

"So get un-used to it because I am going to make you blonde." said Jean.

And so he did.

After that, until the recent assassination attempt on my hair follicles, I had Lauren Bacall blonde hair with highlights. Blunt cut with bangs. It looked super. Especially with the facelift.

So when, in the Capillary Institute, I looked at myself in the mirror wearing the semi-blonde Armanda wig, it perked me right up. Armanda made me look as though I had my own hair again. I wanted to buy it right then and there.

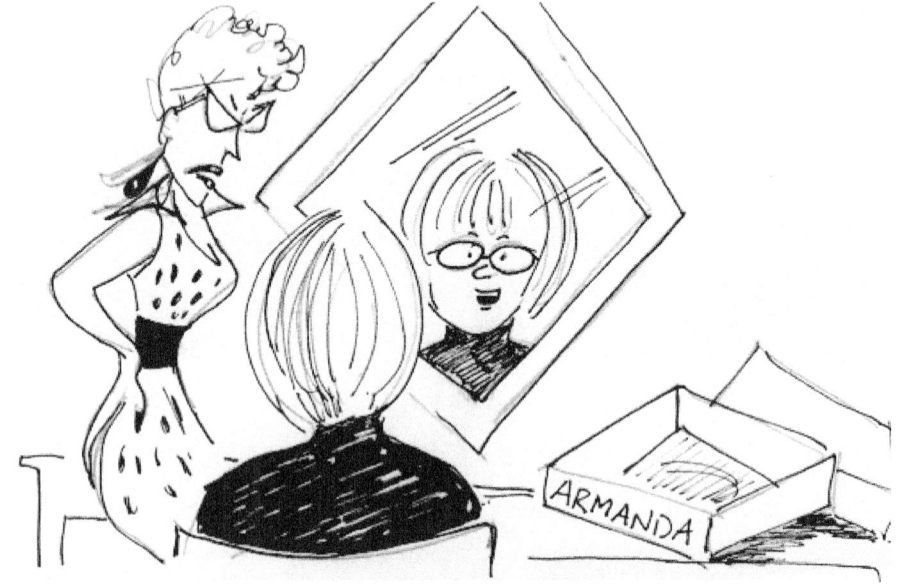

"You ought to try the Patty," Danièle advised. "I think it will suit you better."

I gave Danièle a discreet once over. Too thin. That nervous kind of thin. Fragile. Hair dyed two colors of blonde. Cut short and tightly curled. Frowsy. High heels. Dangling earrings. Frosty nail polish. Makeup base rivulets in the wrinkles. Rhinestones on the spectacles. I was afraid.

But I agreed to try the Patty. She produced it from a box that she first extricated with two broom handles taped together lengthwise to hold a metallic grasping apparatus. Grocers in white aprons used these in old movies to fetch down sacks of foodstuffs from shelves way up over their heads. The bearded face of an old British boyfriend rose up into my mind's eye. It was Nigel. Nigel Fortenberry. Nigel had taught me about those package grabbers. In the UK they call them "lazy tongs." Danièle's double broom handle tongs were so loosely bonded with aging, cracked Scotch Tape, the word *lazy* seemed appropriate.

She gave the hairpiece a few brisk shakes. Then held the Patty wig puppet-style on her hand, and twirled it, beaming.

The Patty, it turned out, was a variegated blonde ringlet wig made of shiny Barbie doll hair. I was about to protest. But I could see that Danièle wanted to dress my head in a wig the cheesy style of which rivaled her own *coiffure*. To accommodate her, I reached around above my forehead, shoved my fingers under Armanda's elastic band, wrenched the wig I loved off my head and placed it on the small *tablette* under the skew-gee mirror. Danièle rapidly took up her post behind me and worked the Patty down over my stinging scalp.

While your hair is falling out during chemotherapy, your head stings. Pascal had explained the process to me on Saturday. He had pushed aside about fifty swatches of varicolored hair samples to reveal a diagram pasted on the wall showing how hairs disengage from their bulbs. As they die and work their way out of the scalp, they lean like wheat in the wind to one side or the other. Their tilting feels like ten naughty boys pulling your pigtails at once.

The skin hurts to the touch and itches. You can't lay your head on the pillow without flinching.

Once she had settled the Patty onto my skull, Danièle gave the wig's hairs a quick whisk with her black plastic wide-toothed comb and stood back to admire my reflection in the mirror. "*Voilà!*" she squealed in a piercing singsong.

I wish you could have seen her *"Voilà!"* The closest I can come to describing it is a "poodle cut". I remembered poodle cuts from the olden days in the 70s. In order to wear this close-to-the-scalp hairdo, you had to either have naturally curly hair or get a perm. A poodle cut in the 21st century? What a concept. Besides, at 71 and bald, I had no desire to resemble a dog - any dog.

But back in 1976, the publisher of my first Chinese Astrology book thought a poodle cut was just what I needed to be born again. When I had shown up from Paris to be published in New York City, I was still sporting the *Parisienne sophistahippy* look. Back then, all hip young French women wore the same outfit with varying tops and footwear: Tight Levis 501 jeans and work shirts or clingy t-shirts and no bra with Frye Boots. Long, straight hair in relative disarray. Real gold earrings and a fake Cartier tank watch.

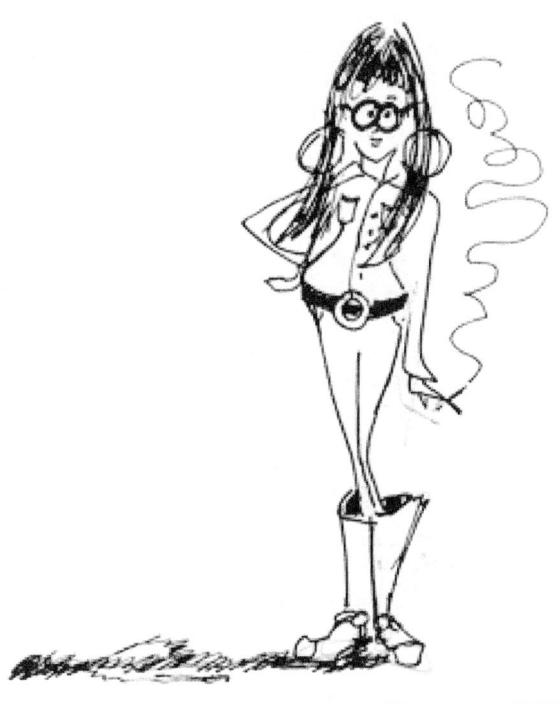

The conservative New York publishers enforced a permanent, a poodle cut and a standard issue Bloomingdale's wardrobe. The photo on the dust jacket of *CHINESE CHANCE* portrayed me as a middle aged, middle class pearls and twin-set woman. A serious Poodle of a woman that a hardback book buyer could believe in. A sensible woman who — even though she writes about some cockamamie animal *oogah boogah* system — is an elegant solid citizen. When the permanent grew out, I let my hair grow long again and reverted to *sophistahippy*.

Danièle couldn't have known about my poodle cut past. But she was dead serious about the look she had in mind for her version of *Madame* White. She really meant it with this Patty Poodle cut plastic hairstyle. *"C'est si feminin,"* she remarked. *"Joli joli."* So feminine. So pretty.

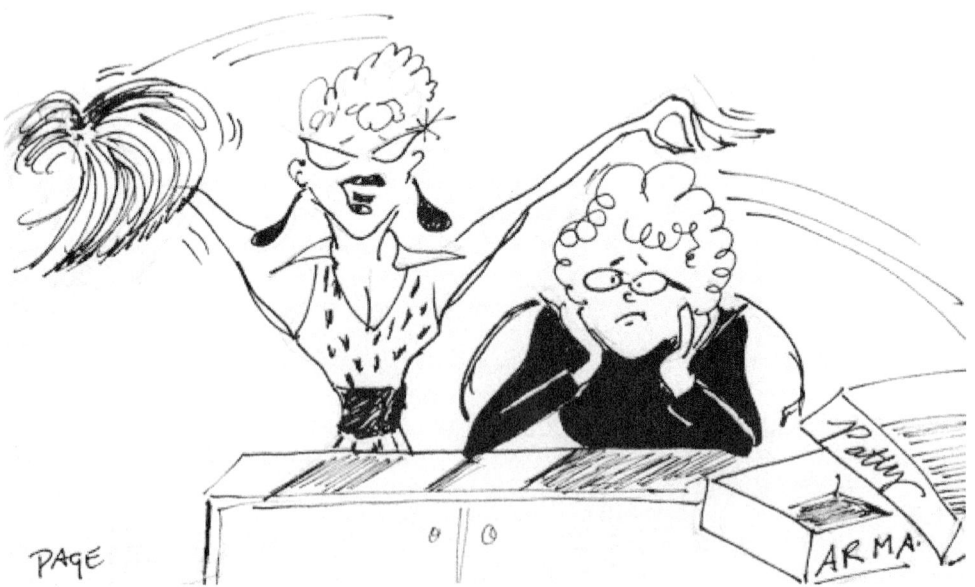

I looked up into the mirror and saw her face. She was glowing. I wanted to puke. It wasn't the chemo. It was the Patty. It resembled a latter day Lucille Ball hairdo with bi-color blonde instead of tight red curls. Lucy Arnaz had an animated, narrowish face with angles. I have a broad flat face — like an English muffin. I wear glasses. Patty and I were a mismatch. Under Patty, my head at top and in back seemed to come to a point. It really looked like a wig. I felt panicky. The way you feel when you leave the hairdresser, race home and stick your head under the faucet. "Danièle, this doesn't work for me," I said.

"But it's lovely on you. You at least look coiffed. With the Patty you will be all the time coiffed."

Me? Coiffed? Jamais. Never.

Being from a family of sales people, it fleetingly occurred to me that the Patty might garner Danièle a higher commission than the Armanda. "What's your astrological sign?" I asked. Mere Sun signs can tell astrologers a lot about a person.

"*Poissons,*" she replied, with a grin. *Pisces.*

"The year?" I inquired.

"1952," she said, fluttering her false eyelashes. Danièle most certainly thought she looked younger than 1952. She wanted me to tell her how terrific she looked for her age. I did not.

Pisces/Dragon Thought I. *A helluva conflict going on in that poodle head.* Once I know a person's "New Astrology" sign, I know approximately how to deal with them. What's New Astrology? It's a system of character reading that I cooked up years ago and wrote a book about. I blended western and Chinese Astrology signs and came up with 144 NEW characters. Some "New Astrology" signs are easier to identify than others. I am a Scorpio/Tiger, an energetic wanderer who cherishes her independence, I get along best with Taurus/Horses, Cancer/Dogs and Pigs, Aries and Capricorn/Roosters and a few Libras of the Horse or Dog variety. But Pisces/Dragons are not easy for me. Pisces tend to be spacey and indecisive. Dragons are often bossy and always need to be right. How I wished Danièle was not a Pisces/Dragon. If only she could have been a Horse or a Dog. At least she would have been on my wavelength.

Imprisoned as my head was under this thoroughly unsuitable fright wig named *Patty*, I actually experienced *hair hunger.* I craved that pretty Armanda non-wiggish wig in the worst way. Armanda's neat, straight hair. My natural color without the white. Nothing fancy. Just Armanda and me. But for some reason, this Pisces/Dragon had more exotic plans for my head. Danièle whisked away the Patty, lay her atop Armanda on the *tablette* before me, grabbed the Josette and started fitting it down over my thin brush cut. *What next?* thought I.

"This one will give you some length," she assured me. "And it has fetching highlights."

This one — the Josette — was black. No blends. Just bluish black. With streaks. Great Zebra platinum bands of whiteish blonde. "The way this one is cut," said Danièle, "it will hide your ears and conceal the rims of your glasses." She swiped the glasses off my face, then put them back on by sliding the rims cunningly into Josette's forest of stringy straight hair. "See?" she said.

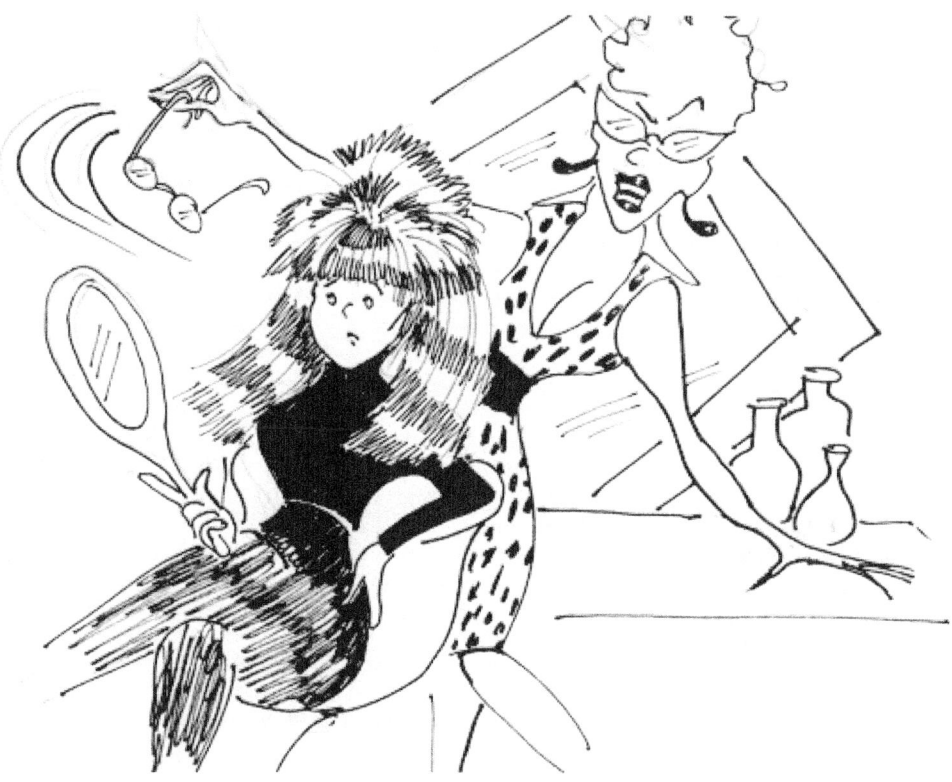

I saw. With Josette on my head, I looked like a well worn Madame whose brothel had gone south. Josette was, in itself, a ridiculous hairstyle. Longer toward the back, bushy layered in front with these platinum stripes! Nobody who was not headed to a masquerade ball would have sported such a rug.

Why was I putting myself through this ordeal? Did I really need a wig? Couldn't I just wear bandanas the way I did the first time I had chemotherapy? *Well, Suze...* said my inner reasonable senior citizen self. *Back then you were 39 and cute and you wore size 8 jeans. Bandanas on pudgy 71 year-old bald ladies? I don't think so.*

This was not my first chance at cancer, so I was somewhat inoculated against the rigors of the treatments. In 1978, two years after the death of my sister Sally from breast cancer, I found a lump on my right breast. Sally's first breast lump had popped up in 1973. Because it hurt, she was convinced it was not cancerous. She went to her neighborhood gynecologist who told her not to worry. It was probably a cyst. Six months later, she had a biopsy and a mastectomy. A year after that she had a second mastectomy. She espoused Christian Science. Opted out of chemotherapy. And even though her arms throbbed with hot pain, she braved the rigors of learning to play tennis. She gave lavish parties and played the guitar. She sang and painted her marvelous paintings with her usual vigor. By the time her doctor convinced her to allow chemotherapy, it was too late for him to save her life. I still weep when I think about losing my brave soldier of a sister. Tears become sobs whenever I flash on the still-grieving copper-haired kids she left behind. Her artistic talent was huge. Her paintings hang in art museums. I knew I would miss her until I died.

Right about then it looked as though I wouldn't be missing Sally for too much longer. I fully expected I was next in line to die. My family history is strewn with women's bodies felled by breast cancer. The Manhattan breast specialist advised me to have a radical mastectomy and one year of chemotherapy. I complied. Back in 1978, chemotherapy drugs were fierce. They were not administered slowly through an intravenous drip. Each month, I drove 25 miles to a hematologist's office. He shot the poisons directly into my arm. Then I got in my car to drive myself home, stopping along the way to heave my cookies out the window. I had pains everywhere.

No hair anywhere. No eyebrows. No pubic hair or leg or arm or underarm hair. A skinned rabbit. My complexion went green and I threw up everything everywhere. When I look back, I do recall buying a wig. But I never wore it much. I used those different colored bandanas.

During that time, I had a fling with a British film director named Robin. He had lost his wife to cancer and was touched by my situation. I liked him and his brain. He spoke about writing and filmmaking and was very gentle and romantic in bed. I got up at 5 in the morning at his house to jump in the car and get home to relieve the overnight babysitter by 6 am so she could get to work on time. After I dressed, I looked back. Robin was sleeping soundly. Next to his head on my pillow writhed giant snarl of my own dark brown hair. It had come out during our lovemaking. I scooped it all up with my fingers and shoved it into my purse. Then I dug around as I drove, found it and threw it out the window on Montauk Highway in Bridgehampton.

That first cancer incident happened in Long Island, USA. I had two perky, pretty small daughters, a sizzling book contract for an epic novel and a brand new house in the dazzling Hamptons. A month later, home from New York Hospital and ready to start my chemotherapy, I received a plain vanilla post card in the mail. It was from Blue Cross, my health Insurance company. It said simply, "Contract # 12870760 has been cancelled." I blinked, gulped and read it again. Looked like Blue Cross/Blue Shield of New York State was canceling my health insurance policy. Why? Because I had cancer? I didn't know and I couldn't find out. Blue Cross would answer neither phone calls nor certified letters.

I was used to living in France with my kids. Over there, I had always worked and paid into the national health system. When we were ill, the health services took care of us. But now we were in the States. Different ball game. I called the Suffolk County social services to ask for help. They asked me if I owned my house. I said yes. They said, "You need to sell it."

And sell it I did. Moved myself and two frightened little girls into a small apartment, changed their schools and used the tiny profit from the house to pay for one year of ferocious chemotherapy. What about the $50,000 worth of outstanding hospital bills that Blue Cross had left me holding the bag for? As soon as my arms were free of needles and I had stopped puking, we packed all the t-shirts and teddy bears and split back to France where we had always lived before.

I don't mean to minimize the impact of this past year's chemotherapeutic episode, but when the surgeon told me I would have six treatments over four months, I was relieved. This time, at least, I was in France. My government health insurance was paid up. Among 31 other illnesses, cancer is considered a serious disease and is covered 100 percent by the French national health care system. My operation, hospitalization, anesthesiologist, drugs, surgeon, nursing care, scans, MRIs and six weeks in a lovely convalescent clinic were paid for by my government health insurance. Oh, and I forgot, physiotherapy and ambulance transport to and from the hospital, as well. Of course I fully realized and was alarmed that I did once again have cancer. That I might die. But this time, at least, I would not be cancelled.

Now Danièle was fussing with another box. I could only see the first letters of that wig's name. Danièle glanced my way, "Oh, you don't like the Josette?"

"It's just not me Danièle. The Armanda is more *me*."

"Well I didn't know you before, did I?" Danièle snapped as she extracted yet another wig from a box the name of which continued to elude my line of sight. "How can I know what is *you*?"

"You can't. But I do know what is *me*. I think the Armanda will do *me* just fine."

"Personally, I find the Armanda dull." said Danièle. She extracted Armanda from under the furry pile on the shelf before me and shook it out. "Look." she said twirling Armanda on her hand. "This wig has no style. None. It's just hair."

"That's what I like about it." I told her. "It's just hair."

Directly after I said that, Danièle tossed the Armanda onto her unruly stack of wigs that looked like a pile of copulating guinea pigs. She then presented me with a new number.

"We call this one the Marilyn," said she, as she thrust a full-blown long blonde wing on my head and then set about fluffing it and bringing the curls forward around my neck. Somehow, if those ears of mine were covered up and the glasses camouflaged, Danièle could once again find me *jolie jolie.* I looked a sight.

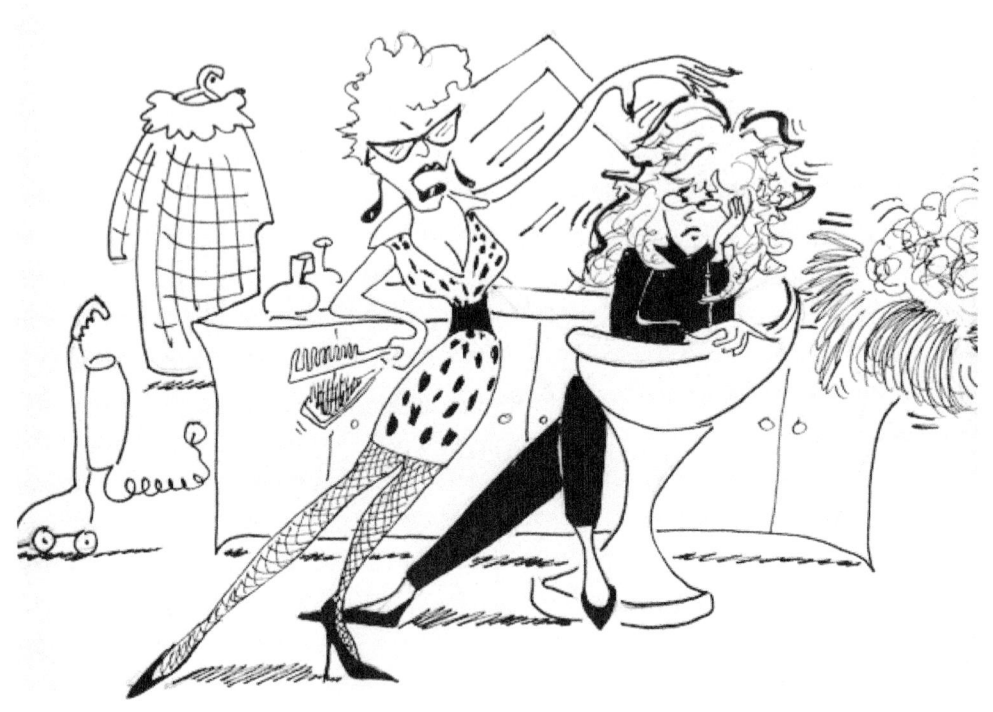

"This one is silly," I told her. "Please remove it."

She yanked it off, leaving me to gaze in the mirror at a spiny-scalped 71-year-old woman with glasses askew. Worse, the way my remaining spikes pointed straight up, I looked like *Tintin* gone bald. I wanted to, but I didn't laugh. It was urgent I remain serious. I had to get out of there with Armanda and back to the *clinique* on time.

Earlier, when I heard I was going to have chemo, Betsy had called me at the *clinique* from Carcès. Betsy's my friend from San Francisco who is here in Provence on sabbatical with her husband Ken. They have a house here. "A wig? How cool is that?" squealed Betsy. "Listen Suze," she went on. "Why not get something bright red and startling? Like a sort of modified Harpo Marx." Betsy is Texas born and bred. A party animal.

"Bets," I replied. "I honestly don't think this is the moment to draw attention to myself with a red wig."

Betsy caught my drift and chilled. But I now realized that Danièle had not. She headed my way with her next number - the Colette. "Danièle," I tried. "I think I can manage with Armanda."

Danièle covered my head with this bouncy curly beige thing with gray highlights. "This one," she said, "is called *'La Colette.'* Like the famous writer."

Mentally, I pictured Colette from old photos I'd seen in her museum house in *Saint Sauveur* in Burgundy. The real Colette had naturally curly gray hair blurred by cigarette smoke. Why did I feel helpless to stop this dervish of nervous energy from playing dress-up with my already too fragile appearance? As she tugged the Colette down around my chin and coaxed errant hairs over my ears, Danièle said, "That husband of mine is a fool. We are married 23 years and he ups and leaves me."

Uh Oh. Now I was in for it. My whole morning would be devoured by this addled, bossy creature. I would not make it to the pharmacy for my herbal shampoo before noon when everything in sight in France closes for the ritual two-hour lunch. Instead, I would surrender to the wiles of Danièle, the flakey wig monger. For the next hour and some minutes, I would try on the Jeanette (layered, chin length auburn with strident whitish tips) and the Diane, (subtle salt and pepper, pompadour in front, blackish stringy in back), the Marie-France, (short, upside-down artichoke with golden tipped leaves), the Gloria (blonde, long *Farah Fawcettesque*), and others. I politely rejected every one of Danièle's fantasy disguises.

But I was fuming inside. And plotting. *How can I kidnap Armanda and take her home with me?*

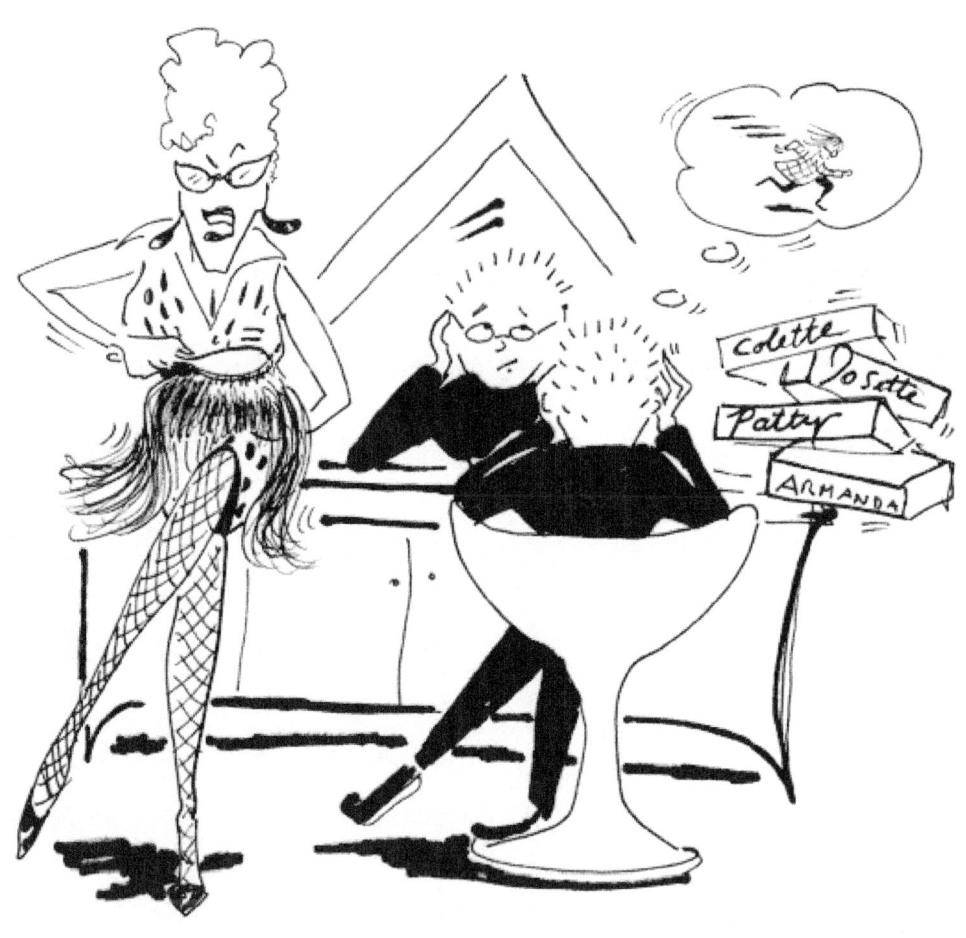

My head was nearly shorn bald. I needed to be back at the convalescent *clinique* by lunchtime, which is noon sharp. It takes 20 minutes to drive there. I had to abscond with Armanda right away.

Without her, it would be awkward. I didn't fancy breaking bread bald with my three broken-hipped tablemates. They had lived through the war years. They knew what a *tondue* looked like. Collaborator women's faces would flash through their minds for sure. My brain saved me. *Change the subject,* it advised.

As she was snuggling the Denise (wig #10) down over my aching cranium, I tried, "How much does the Armanda cost, please?"

She stopped mid yank and scurried from the room, leaving me sitting there with the fluffy Denise aslant over my right cheek. "I'll go check," said her disappearing voice.

In a minute Danièle returned, reading from a large catalogue. "It looks like 529 euros," she muttered, tracing her finger down a row of small print figures. She threw a look at me agape, dropped the catalogue to the floor and exclaimed, *"Oh la la. Oh Madame White. Oh Pardon. Oh la la."*

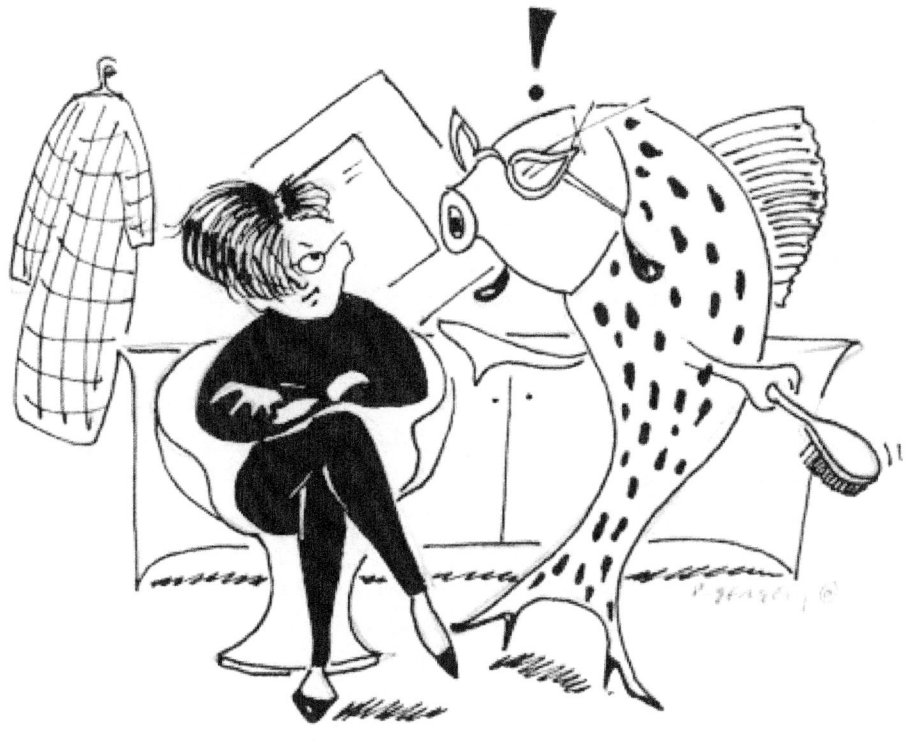

Typical Pisces. Lost in a dream, snaps awake and notices I am half in - half out of her *Denise*. Now she is sorry. Begging my forgiveness. "It's my divorce," she explained. "I am next to my shoes." This folkloric French expression means "I am out of sorts," which, for my money, in English, is equally opaque. What are sorts and how come we run out of them?

While she was arranging the hairs of the pixie cut Denise (Audrey Hepburn, age 28) atop my head, I asked, "Was the divorce your idea or his?"

She stopped mid comb and said, "His."

The heap of exotic guinea pigs – that pile of sadly rejected hairpieces on the counter beneath the skew gee mirror – was all but laughing at me.

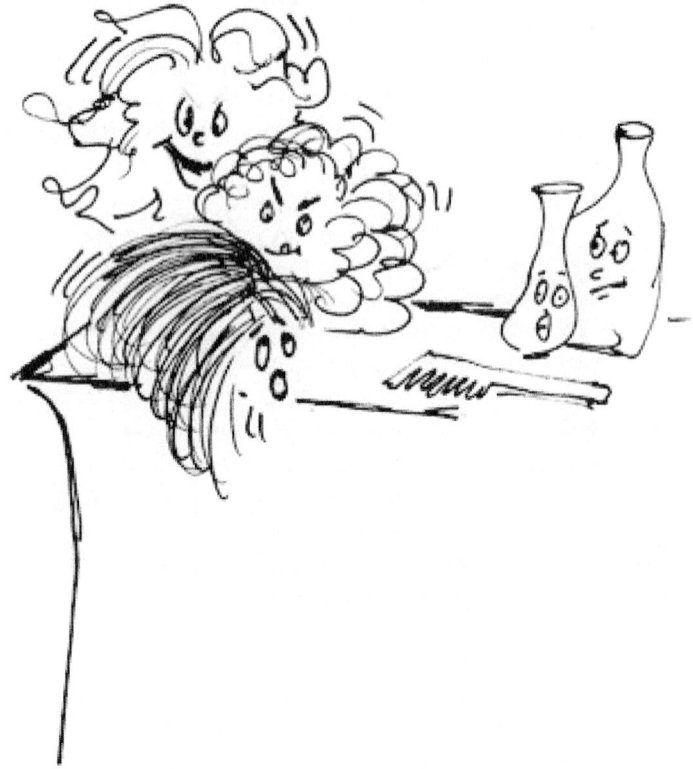

How many wigs, I worried, will it take for her to spill me her whole divorce story? Why did I ask?

She urged three more wigs on me. It was coming on 11:15. I had to be back at *Les Espérels.* "He decided to leave me. It's about money. We were married for 23 years. How can he do this to me?"

"Maybe there's someone else," I suggested.

"MY husband? With another woman? Impossible. He isn't even interested in sex," said Danièle.

"Really?" I wondered. "Then why would he leave?"

"He says he's tired of Provence. He wants to live in Brittany. Near the sea," Danièle said. "He's *Breton.* They are a race apart. I don't trust them. He's lucky I married him. New genes with that rotten *Breton* blood."

Mmmhhhh. I thought. *This Dragon lady has some fire left in her snout.* Meanwhile I figure that Papa's got himself a comely *Bretonne* up there in Oysterland by the beautiful sea and wants to rip off my wiggy friend Danièle's last *centîme.* I was about to lament his departure with her when she asked how I felt about the perky, shellacked Denise.

"This is really not my style," I replied. "I still like the Armanda."

Danièle was having none of it. She said, "Pascal mentioned, Madame White, that you are an *astrologue.*"

Oh no. Not here. Not now. I knew it. She's going to want me to tell her fortune.

Command performance… Out of the blue! Pascal ratted me out. I was captive. Here! Hairless! In this palace of dinge and plaster dust, I was going to be astro-interrogated by this flibbertigibbet. "I dabble in astrology," I muttered, hoping to throw her off.

"But... but... Pascal said you are *famous.*"

I looked up at Danièle. "I don't really know very much about astrology," I said. "I sort of fake it."

"But you *are* famous. Pascal said so. He said you are a *famous* Astrology writer from America." Danièle slathered me with an ingratiating smile and sort of shimmied at the same time.

"May I just buy the Armanda please?" I begged.

"I met somebody." Danièle whispered. "He's a Taurus. Why do I always end up with Tauruses?"

Oh God please give me strength. If I let Danièle's love life seem to matter for one split second, Armanda and I might be washed up. The doctor had only granted me a morning's leave to see to my headgear. I had to be back. "Maybe you are attracted to earthy types," I remarked.

"They are sexy," she said. "Once, last year though, I had a Scorpio after me."
She skittered around behind me and went on. "He came to prune the trees.
Then he would not leave me alone. I explained there was someone else. But
he persisted. I had to get nasty."

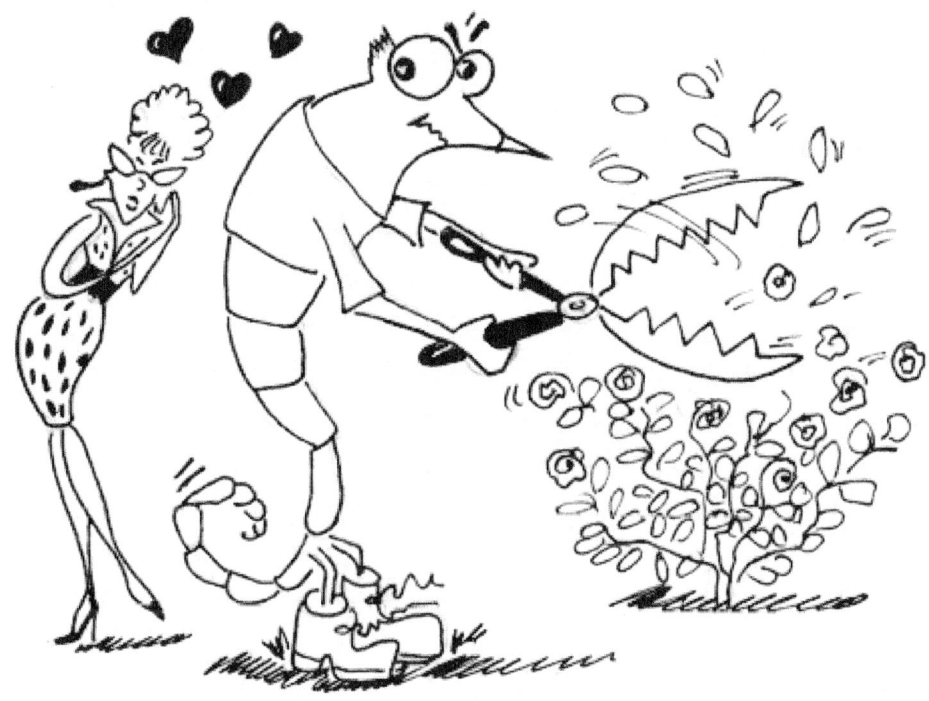

"Oh really?"

"He was *furieux* with me. He said I had led him on. I mean, I was nice to
him, Madame White. It was hot outside. I invited him in for a beer,"
Danièle continued. "But I did not make advances to him." Danièle tisked

like a pro. "I swear Madame White, he was close to violence. No more Scorpios in my garden. They insist way too much. I mean, he was attractive. But I told him. I already had somebody."

I hit fast forward. "I need to go now," I blurted. "Pascal told me on Saturday to leave him a check. He said he wouldn't cash it till the government health insurance and the anti-cancer league pay me for their participation."

The phone rang. Danièle scurried into the other room to answer. I wrenched Denise off my head, clapped on Armanda and grabbed my coat and purse. Checkbook in hand, I exited the wig room and entered the office cubicle. When she got off the phone I handed Danièle my check for 529 euros. "I am going now," I said.

"Pascal told me you write books."

I know this trick. Flattery. Groveling. Anything to make me stay here and dissect her divorce saga.

"What kind of books?"

"Books about animals." I said, tossing my loose new locks nonchalantly.

"Wild animals," I added. *Au revoir.* See you again sometime."

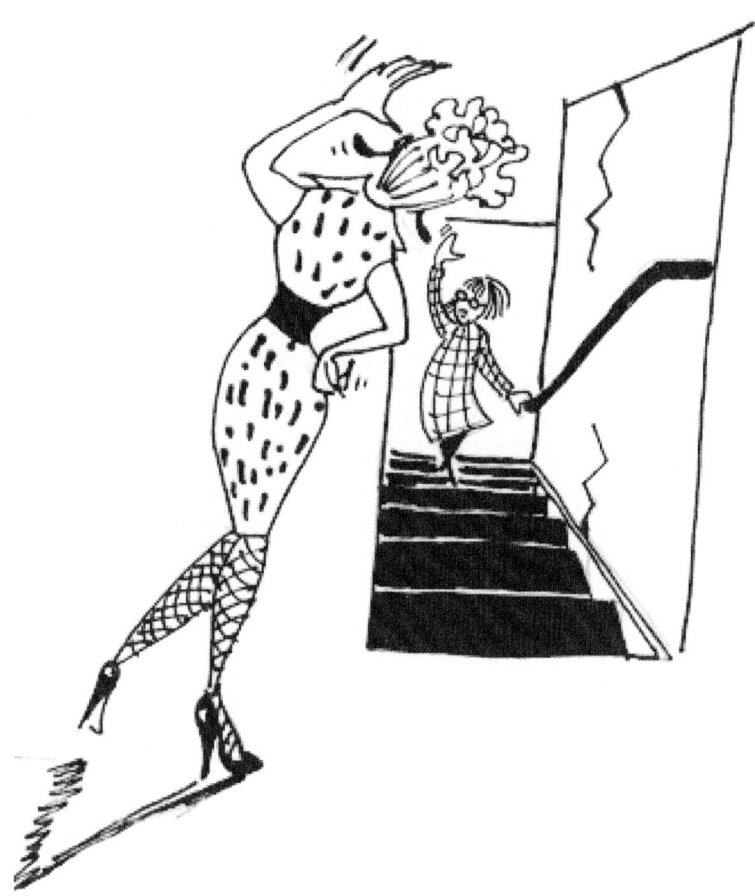

I picked my way down the Capillary Institute's dark, treacherous staircase and ran along the street to Jean's *salon de coiffure*. As I said earlier, Jean is a blabbermouth. But he's still the best. I needed his aesthetic approval. As I pushed open the door to his salon, Jean saw me from afar. "*Parfait!*" He exclaimed. In French "*parfait*" doesn't mean ice cream sundae. It means "perfect." Made my day.

I clutched Armanda to my aching scalp and raced to the car. It was twelve to twelve. I drove like hell on the twisty roads and got back just in time for my lunch, which had already been served in the *clinique's* restaurant. I delivered the ritual *Bonjour Mesdames* to one and all, sat right down and began to eat my endive salad *hors d'oeuvre*. We all chatted. Some noticed the wig. And some did not. Nobody said a thing.

After the cheese course, the eldest lady at the table squinted across at me. "Have you been to the hairdresser?" she asked.

 I nodded yes.

"I thought your hair looked longer," she said, and chomped the end off her *éclair au chocolat*.

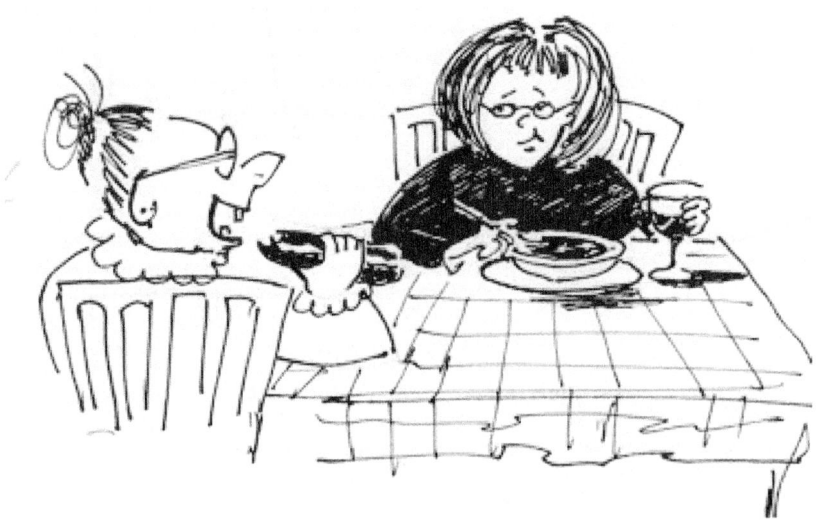

the end/ fin

More Books by Suzanne White

CHINESE ASTROLOGY PLAIN AND SIMPLE

A complete, easy-to-use guide to the Chinese horoscope. This ancient zodiac system is based on a cycle of twelve years, each governed by a particular animal. Each of us has an animal sign. Our destiny and character depend on it. This book provides startling insights into your friends, lovers and yourself. Peppered throughout are anecdotes about famous personalities, illustrating how their characters are influenced by their birth years.

THE NEW ASTROLOGY

A worldwide best-seller, The New Astrology is a massive undertaking. There are not 12 but 144 signs of the New Zodiac. Each of us is governed by two signs. Chinese and Western. Suzanne White shows us how to better understand ourselves and others. She's lucid, amusing yet serious. This lifetime reference book explains everything about everyone you know - including yourself!

THE NEW CHINESE ASTROLOGY

Here we are generously exposed to the full gamut of Chinese Astrology. Suzanne White offers voluminous descriptions of the twelve animals, then further divides them into sixty by adding the five key elements. She gives a future outlook for all signs up to the year 2020. The book is over 500 pages long. Some Chinese Astrology books are "cute." Some take themselves deadly serious. This book is versatile. It's also hard-hitting. The author doesn't believe in pulling punches. Whether your Chinese sign is egotistical or wimpy, you will hear about it in this jolly, informative volume by world famous author/astrologer Suzanne White.

THE ASTROLOGY OF LOVE
(The Matchmaker's Guide to the Universe)

Don't get married or move in with anyone until you own this essential couples guide book. Suzanne White has matched all 24 astrological signs (Chinese and western) and come up with accurate, practical and humorous results. A Dragon born Taurus might very well get along with a Monkey born in Cancer. But if you are a Scorpio born in a Tiger year, there is not much hope for you with a Gemini born Goat. White defines each coupling with heart scores. 4 hearts = Bed of Roses 3 Hearts = Bed & Breakfast 2 hearts = Breakfast in Bed 1 heart = pillow fights. And Zero hearts = Bed of Nails! Get this book BEFORE you fall into the tender trap.

LADYFINGERS (A NOVEL) 1975

A young American woman's search for the perfect orgasm leads her to elegant Paris where she encounters a wealthy Californian Prince Charming who turns out to be the perfect Prince of Darkness. She has two baby princesses with her barefoot lord and master, then discovers he has no money. She escapes from Paris back to Buffalo, New York with both babies and impoverished Prince in tow. There, in the dingy rustbelt American city, the idle Prince's sheep's clothing wears rapidly thin. The young woman finds an unusually adventurous solution to the problem.

All Books Available on Paper at Major Booksellers.

E-book for sale on Kindle

Free Horoscopes, Personal Chart Readings and Astrological Advice

at http://www.suzannewhite.com

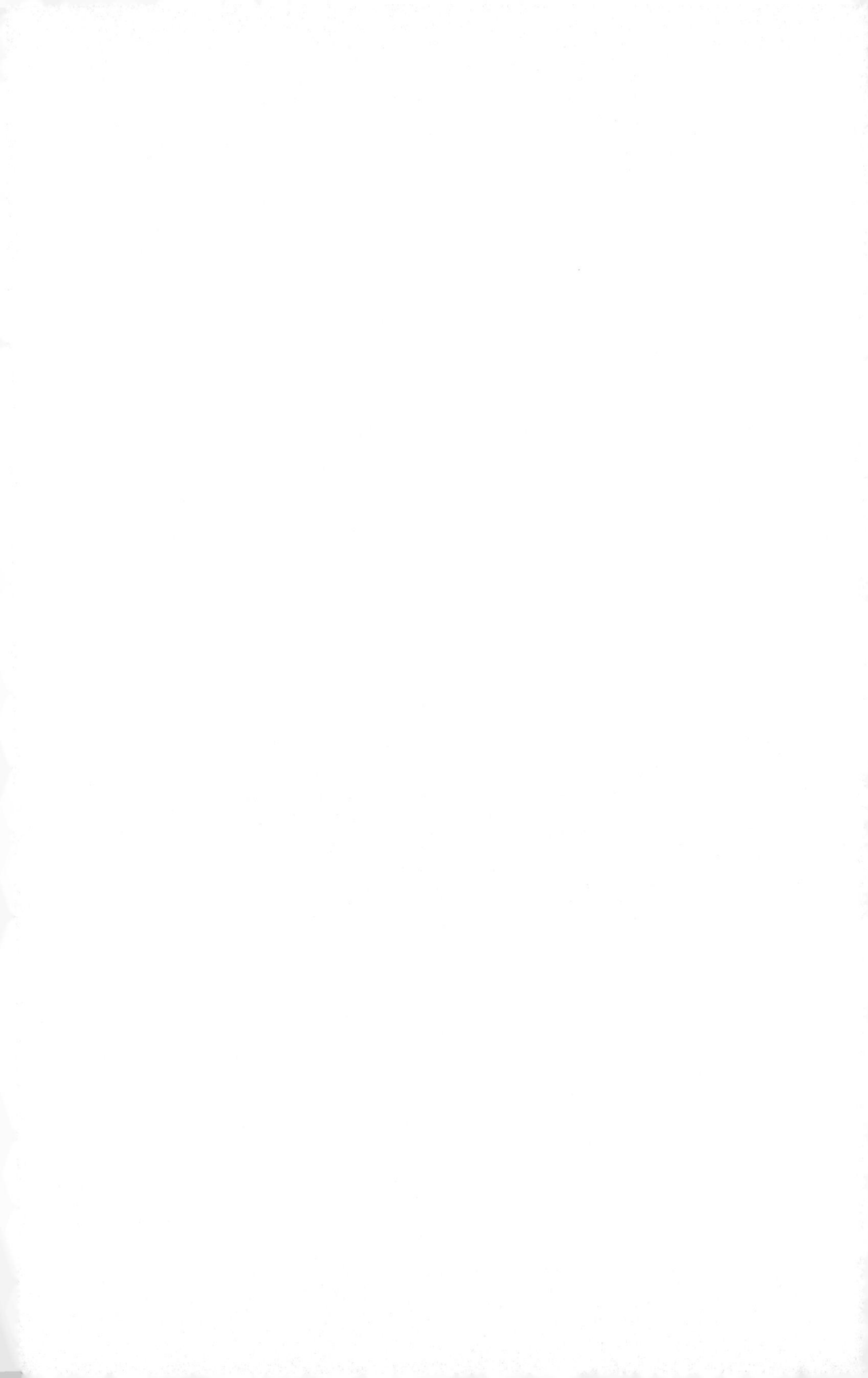

Printed in Great Britain
by Amazon

65824966R00031